Eczema Cure Today

Get rid of Eczema forever, natural ways to cure Eczema

Smit Chacha

© Copyrighted 2017

978-1-387-30798-2
Imprint: Lulu.com

http://www.eczemacuretoday.com/

Introduction

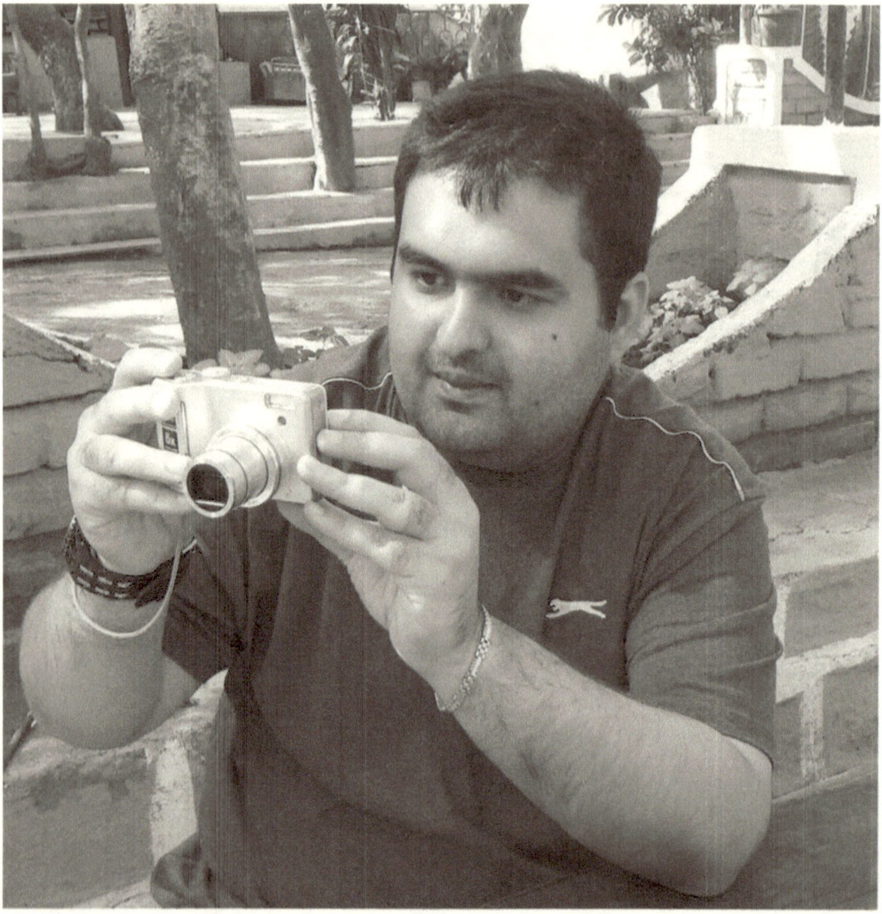

Hi,

My name is Smit Chacha and I am the author of this book. I have been writing and publishing articles in several subjects (including Eczema) all over the internet as an EzineArticles Expert Author:

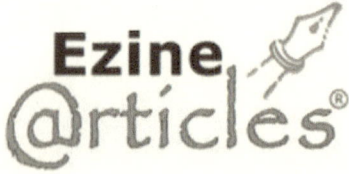

https://ezinearticles.com/expert/Smit_Chacha/

I do not possessed any degree or qualifications in medicine. I do however possessed a Bsc. Degree in Computer Visualization and Games.

For the past 10 years I have been writing and publishing articles all over the web, promoting other people stuff as an online affiliate marketer.

Why did I published this book?

After 10 years of writing and promoting other people stuff, I found myself in a position to start publishing my own books. I have wrote over 400 articles in this niche (Eczema).

This book contains the essential guide to treat and cure Eczema at home. It is full with my top tips thoroughly researched and published as an EzineArticles Expert Author.

I hope you will enjoy reading it…..

Smit Chacha

Table of Contents

Eczema Cure Today - get rid of eczema forever, natural ways to cure eczema

Eczema is an ugly skin disease that causes severe itchiness, pain and a very uncomfortable felling! This outrageous skin disorder can happen to anyone at any time, from young children to more mature people.

This skin disease is so painful and get even worse if it is not treated, as you can see below:

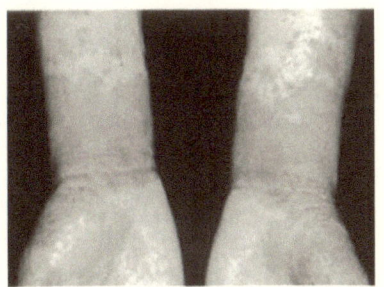 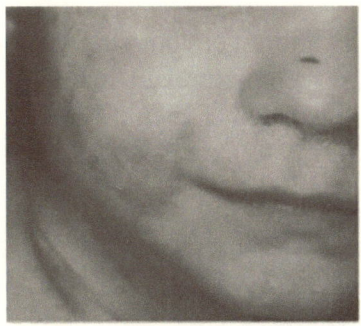

If you are experiencing an intense itching feeling that just won't go away, no matter how strongly you scratch. **Then you probably got Eczema!**

If certain foods, fabrics, cosmetics, soaps and even stress causes your skin to be irritated **then you probably got Eczema!**

Whenever you suffer deep stinging sensations and your skin slowly oozes blood and white sticky pus. **Then you probably got Eczema!**

Beware! If your skin doesn't begin to self-renew or self-repair no matter what you do and things are getting bad to worse. **Then you might find yourself with severe eczema!**

But finally there is a solution! A natural and organic solution that will heal your Eczema problems in matter of 10 days or less! As seen on the pictures below:

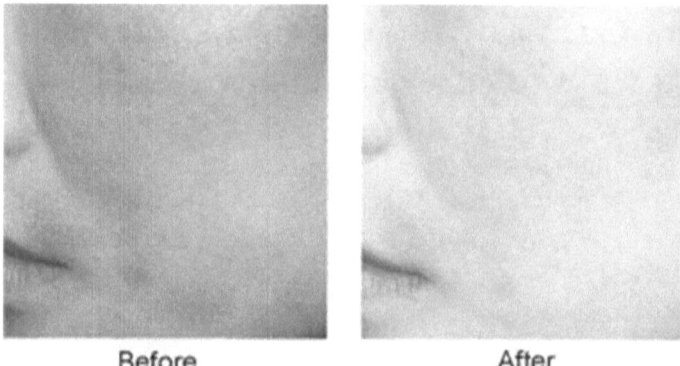

Before   After

If you want to get your skin smoother, healthier and Eczema free just like the seen picture above, then I strongly recommend that you read this Book titled "Eczema Cure Today – get rid of eczema for ever, natural way to cure eczema"

Eczema Disease

Eczema is an angry looking skin condition, which can look dry, scaly, itchy and inflamed. In most countries, 1 in 5 children suffers from eczema and 1 in 12 adults are living with some degree of this condition.

You may be given antihistamine medication to make your skin less itchy. This should also help you to sleep better at night by reducing itching.

Vitamin C and Vitamin F are often helpful in hydrating skin from the inside out.

Many Eczema sufferers scratch whilst sleeping if you do scratch your Eczema whilst asleep try wearing some thin cotton gloves to bed this should stop you from scratching and causing any more damage to your skin.

Gotu Kola is said to be a good Herb to help ease the itchiness with people who have Eczema look for a cream or tincture that contains this ingredient if you have trouble finding something suitable look for creams or tinctures containing Camomile, Witch Hazel or Liquorice as these all reduce skin inflammations or irritations.

The severity of your skin condition will determine how long you have to take the medication. The more severe it is, the shorter the period of time because you may soon suffer from serious side effects such as vascular necrosis of the hip

But there is another way you can get relief or even cure eczema. And this does not require any medicine, it is totally organic and natural.

I am talking about organic medicine that involves consuming fruits and vegetables. Fruits and vegetables are naturally rich in vitamins and minerals that give natural relief from eczema.

Eczema - Definition and Treatment

Eczema is a kind of disease characterized by skin inflammation. Atopic dermatitis, is the most common form of eczema, which leads to chronic, recidivating and very itchy rash's on the skin. Infants are the most vulnerable although it can attack people of any age group. The National Institute of Health predicted that almost 10 to 20 percent of infants are infected. This can also occur because of hereditary problems, but mostly due to the abnormal behavior of the body's immune system, which are triggered by some irritable substances and allergens in the environment.

Although Atopic Dermatitis is the most usual form of Eczema, it has a variety of patterns. Some of them are named as: Contact Eczema, Seborrheic Eczema, Nummular Eczema, Neuro Dermatitis, Stasis Dermatitis and Dyshydrotic Eczema. Each one is characterized by their specific symptoms. But dry, red, inflamed, itchy and burning skins are the most common symptoms in all forms despite its diverse appearance from person to person.

Even though there is no complete cure, Eczema is not contagious. But it is so virulent that a patient cannot ignore itching which triggers him to scratch and get things worse. The victim should detect the root cause of the problem which may be due to lack of nutrients, the action of allergens or some malfunctioning of the body.

The most advisable way to prevent and get rid of this dangerous illness is to adopt a healthy lifestyle. The victim should modify his/her lifestyle based on the root cause. Allergens, if detected should be completely prohibited. Acidity may also be one of the causes. So, the patient should change to a diet which has more alkali. Eating raw vegetables and fruits in the morning, can provide nearly 65% of calories needed, and is the best way to eliminate Eczema. Fruits and vegetables, the highest nutrient storehouse of all foods, contains Phytonutients which also helps to remove the toxins even at the cellular level.

How Does Eczema Look Like?

Eczema is a skin disease that causes rashes; it is a very irritating and uncomfortable disease. Eczema tends to give a reddish pigment to the skin, which is called rash. This rash is very irritating and itchy; it also tends to dry out the skin very quickly. This is the reason why people with eczema tend to moisturize their skin so often, they tend to use creams to alleviate the "pain" as well as to moisturize the skin and to rebuild the skin dry out.

But what most people do not know is that creams are artificially enhanced with 2 vital nutrients, but these nutrients (vitamin E and Aloe Vera). These 2 nutrients are the fuel source of the skin defense system.

What people should know is that many fruits and vegetables also offer these nutrients for Free, so why take them artificially and spend thousands of dollars on creams if we can give our skin the nutrients that they need on fruits and vegetables!

Below are some of the fruits that you should eat to receive these rich nutrients and help your skin to fight against eczema:

- Blackberries
- Avocado
- Plums
- Almonds
- Hazel nuts
- Peanuts
- Broccoli
- Leeks
- Spinach
- Potato

I also would like to add one more tip. Try to wear cotton clothes instead of wool, because wool tends to provoke eczema, and this often results in a quick spread of the disease. But the cotton do the exact opposite, cotton has been proven to ease the itchiness of eczema, try for yourself and you will see the difference instantly.

What Causes Eczema

What is the cause of eczema?

There are many factors that contribute the spread of this disease. The most common is the constant scratching. The simple act of scratching helps the disease to multiply and spread their way further to your skin. So no matter how itchy and irritating eczema get, please do not scratch!

Another reason is the use of wool cloths; wool is a very good conductor of this disease. If you wear wool cloths you will find your skin so irritating that it will turn your skin color to red. So avoid wearing wool cloths instead wear cotton wear. Cotton as been proven to be a very itchy free material, why? Because cause is a very soft cloth and also a worm material. So from now of, wear lots of cotton wear, and you will see the difference on your itchiness.

The third is the most common cause, moisturizing. You must moisturize your skin as often as you can, this will help you skin self-defense system to work properly. The act of moisturizing your skin will clean your skin from bad bacteria and open your skin spurs that will give the passage way for the skin defense system.

Another possibility of causing eczema is an allergic reaction, you see many materials can react with your skin, like wool as I mention before, but there are others such as: pets, dust, perfumes, makeup and detergent. The reason that they react to badly with your skin, is because there use chemicals.

The best way to clean your skin with chemicals is to moisturize your skin, like taking a bath or a shower. Another alternative is to use creams, as most of them uses vitamin E and Aloe Vera, these ingredients are vital for the skin self-defense system. And if you really like to use fragrances, this can be an alternative for you as well, because you can easily find perfumed creams on the shops. Yes they are also made from chemicals, but they also have rich nutrients that are good for your skin health.

What is Eczema exactly? What are the symptoms?

Eczema is not an allergy itself, but allergies can trigger eczema. Some environmental factors (such as excessive heat or emotional stress) can also trigger the condition. Eczema is not infectious and cannot be spread to other people.

Eczema is often very itchy and when you scratch it, the skin becomes red and inflamed. Eczema is simply an external presentation of an internal disorder due to lowered vitality and immunity. When the whole person is treated, the power of immune system is enhanced thereby causing the disease to disappear. Eczema is a symptom not a diagnosis! Eczema is sometimes called dermatitis which means 'inflammation of the skin'. There are different types of eczema.

Babies are especially sensitive to chemical irritants, and sometimes even the slight residue from detergents and fabric softeners will lead to irritation. Dryer-sheet softeners are especially notorious in this regard; even if you are not using them on the baby's clothes, if you use dryer sheets on your own clothes the sheets leave a residue on the inside of the dryer which then comes off on the baby's wash in the next load (the residue can persist for several loads after the sheets are used, as a matter of fact). Babies inevitably want to scratch itchy skin, but you can minimise this by putting on cotton gloves or mittens.

Eczema is treated with moisturizing agents, and if it's severe, may also need to be treated with steroid creams or other prescription ointments. Eczema is worsened when the skin is dry, so oils and moisturising creams applied directly to the skin are helpful, as is the use of bath oils. All these help to prevent the skin from becoming dry.

What Are the Eczema Skin Symptoms?

People frequently ask me "what are eczema symptoms?" this lead me to write an article and hopefully to answer all the common questions that your might have.

Before we answer the question, we must know first what eczema is. Eczema, has most of you should know, is a skin disease that makes the skin irritated and itchy.

Now what are the most common symptoms? Well, we already mention some them, itchiness is the most common symptom it generally makes the skin with a reddish pigment and it is very irritating, some people call it rash skin.

Another common symptom is white pus and comes after red pigment, this doesn't happen to everyone, reason why that pus comes out I do not know.

Dry skin is another common eczema symptom, this is the reason it is so important to moisture your skin constantly when you suffer from eczema.

And finally what makes this disease different from others is that eczema can spread very quickly!

Now to conclude this article I want to share with you some of home remedy that will help you to cure or relief from eczema.

First of all, you must take daily baths or shower, this will clean your skin surface from unwanted bacteria's that are blocking the skin self-defense system to perform the task to fight eczema from down under.

Also you must consume lots of fruits and vegetables that are rich in Vitamin E and Aloe Vera, these 2 nutrients are vital for a healthy looking skin.

And if you suffer from eczema then you must avoid using fragrances, as they provoke the disease and make them spread even quicker throw your body.

Can You 'Catch' Eczema?

Eczema as you know is a skin disease that causes severe itchiness, dryness, irritation, inflammation, redness and sometimes bleeding. But how do you catch eczema?

Well, you can catch this disease by following ways:

Family inheritance: meaning if a direct member of your family is or was diagnosed with dermatitis then you are a highly likely to inherit it.

Allergies: dust, pets and other allergic candidates can easily strike eczema, especially if you have a sensitive skin.

Lack of nutrients: lack of vital nutrients can definitely strike eczema, specially vitamin E and Aloe Vera, these are vital skin nutrients. They are the fuel that maintains our skin healthy and therefore if our body and skin suffers from lack of these vital ingredients your body will react and therefore eczema will appear or strike!

So how can I avoid eczema?

For starters have a regular healthy diet, rich in vitamin E and Aloe Vera. Prevent your body and skin from suffering a lack of these vital nutrients.

Drinking 2/3 liters of water a day is also a good idea, as you know dry skin can strike eczema and one of its symptoms is dryness. Therefore drinking the daily recommend amount of water will prevent this to happen as well as dehydration. If you maintain your body hydrated the chances are the you will not require a constant use of body moisturizers.

Wearing cotton clothes is also a good idea; cotton is a very soft, smooth and itchy free material. Therefore by wearing cotton wear you will reduce skin irritation and therefore eczema.

Avoiding fragrances, detergents and other chemical made products is also advisable. These are made from harsh chemicals that can react very badly specially over a sensitive skin, which can lead to eczema to appear.

Eating healthy dose of fruits such as: apples, bananas, berries, beaches, apricots, mangoes, coconuts, pears and oranges is always a good advice, not only for avoiding eczema but also do avoid many other diseases. Fruits and veggies contain plenty of vitamins and minerals and with a healthy amount of these vital nutrients we drastically reduce our chances of suffering any sort of diseases.

Why Eczema is Normal

Eczema is normal not appear simply because our skin suffers from numerous intruders every day. Things like: weather, dust, allergies, lack of nutrients and even fashion can trigger eczema. In this article I will share some effective ways to avoid and even cure Eczema using only natural and organic products. Eczema is a skin disease that causes itchiness, redness, irritation, inflammation and dryness. This common skin condition is very normal among children, teenagers and adults. There are loads of ways to get infected with Eczema, thing like:

- weather
- dust
- allergies
- lack of nutrients
- fashion

Although there is nothing we can do about weather, but there are some precautions that we can make to the all other things motioned above. Dusk, allergies and fashion (I will get to the lack of nutrients later on) can be easily avoided. Things like detergents, perfumes can easily trigger eczema. These sort of products contain harsh chemicals that react very badly among sensitive skin thus Eczema appear, its normal to this to happen. Believe it or not but clothes can also strike Eczema! Wool for instance can trigger Eczema, wool is a very irritated material and can be allergic and this can easily cause rash. So you see it is normal to have Eczema.

Tip: wear cotton clothes instead, cotton unlike wool is a very soft, smooth and itchy free material. Studies show that cotton upon direct contact with a disease skin (Eczema skin) provides instantaneous relief from its symptoms.

Lack of nutrients, this can be a huge factor. You see our skin requires 2 key nutrients. Vitamin E and Aloe Vera, with a lack of these nutrients Eczema is natural to strike. Therefore it is recommended that you eat fruits and vegetables as often as you can, they contain a high level of these key nutrients. Water is also a factor; you see our body requires water to keep the body and skin moist. With a lack of water our skin can suffer from dehydration causing skin dryness. When that happens Eczema is natural to appear.

So you see Eczema is normal and it can happen to anyone at any time.

Eczema - Can I Really Treat It?

Eczema is actually a disease in a kind of dermatitis, or you can say an inflammation of the epidermis. This term is specifically and widely applied to an array of tenacious skin situations.

These situations include recurring skin rashes and dryness which are featured with one or more these symptoms like bleeding, oozing, cracking, blistering, flaking, crusting, dryness, itching, skin edema that is swelling, or redness.

The regions of temporary skin discoloration may appear and many timed due to the healed lesions. Scratching may open the lesion which may result in scarring. It may also be found on the flexor muscles and joint areas.

The question arises how to cure eczema completely?

You can surely cure eczema through natural ways. If you really use an efficient method for the treatment, then just stick to it. This way you can cure your eczema completely and very soon.

The fact is this how your body reacts to different ways of cure and treatment. To be really loyal, the natural cure is the best cure and a better alternative than the creams and medicines and all. This is because many people's eczema gets worsen after employing the creams and strong medicines. Do not try to get relief on the context of pain.

In a natural way, the following few things are the best things that can cure you completely and provide you permanent relief from eczema:

- Use natural and topical oils like Vitamin D oil, extra virgin olive oil and so on. They bring back the moisture into the skin and eliminate the cracked skin area and dryness in order to provide smoothness and relief.
- Apply the pack of mud on the infected area.
- Oatmeal baths can prove to be really helpful in eliminating the eczema as it makes the skin smooth and stops itching.

Standard Treatment of Eczema Vs Natural Treatment for Eczema

In this article I will reveal the advantages and disadvantages of the standard treatment of Eczema VS the natural and organic treatment for Eczema.

Eczema as you know is a skin disorder that causes itchiness, redness, irritation, inflammation and dryness. This disease is very common among children although recent studies suggest that adults are also very vulnerable.

In this article I will going to show you 2 ways to treat this skin disease. A standard way and an organic way. I will also mention the advantages of using each of them.

Standard Eczema treatment: it's composed from the standard medicines like: creams, lotions and pills. This treatment is very effective fighting Eczema and very assessable, you can find these medicines very easily in almost every chemist. Although there are a few disadvantages of using this treatment. Eczema moisturizers (creams, lotions and pills) tend to be very expensive and some do cause side effects. This pretty much sums up as far as standard Eczema treatment is.

Organic Eczema treatment: this is a more natural approach to fight this skin disease, it's purely made from natural products such as fruits and vegetables that contain a high level of nutrients (vitamin E and Aloe Vera) which are the key for a smooth and healthy skin. (Vitamin E and Aloe Vera is what creams, lotions and pills have, made from chemicals of course). What organic medicine approaches is to consume natural products (fruits and veggies) instead artificially enhanced nutrients (creams, lotions and pills). The biggest advantage of this approach is that is virtually causes zero side effects! And that pretty much sums up as far as organic treatment is. There are no disadvantages.

Treating Eczema without Prescription

You can treat Eczema without prescription, I have nothing against prescribe drugs; they do work however I find that some of them cause several long term side effects. Natural treatments that I am going to reveal to you case absolutely zero negative effects.

Before I jump to the natural ways to treat eczema let me first tell you what prescribe drugs do. These drugs are artificially enhanced with nutrients that reduces eczema symptoms and they are: vitamin E and Aloe Vera.

Having this knowledge you can now treat your eczema naturally! Simply eat healthy foods that are rich in these two nutrients. Fruits and veggies are boosted with vitamins and minerals. My suggestions eat: spinach, grape, plums, peanuts, leeks and broccoli.

Another natural way to treat eczema is by drinking 2 liters of water a day. Dehydration is among the most common cause that triggers eczema, therefore by drinking the daily recommended amount of water you can prevent eczema to strike.

Here is another tip: if you are suffering from several eczema I suggest you wear cotton clothes, cotton is a very smooth, soft and itchy free material and by simply wearing cotton you will notice a drastic reduce in your eczema symptoms.

Ayurveda tips for eczema

The reality is that eczema can be treated without any sort of prescriptions, with a few little lifestyle changes you can drastically reduce eczema symptoms.

What causes eczema? Eczema can be cause from a variety of factors such as: allergies from soaps, detergents, lotions, fragrances, environment you live in, etc. By eliminating certain things you can reduce your chances of reducing this skin disease.

Once you know which of the factors is causing dermatitis you can act accordingly. Most people think that medication is the only way to cure eczema, however this is not true!

Sure, prescribe creams are good to treat this disease, however they are expensive and some can cause side effects. Also, it will not guarantee that eczema will strike again. Below are few lifestyle changes that you can easily implement and you will reduce eczema problems for life.

Avoid wearing scratchy clothes that make you sweat, instead wear cotton clothes. Drink plenty of water a day to moisturize your body and skin. Eat fruits and vegetables that are high in vitamin E and Aloe Vera, these are the body skin vital nutrients that have magical ingredients to fight eczema.

Creams are artificially enhanced with these nutrients via harsh and expensive chemicals that can cause side effects and it will not guarantee that eczema strikes again in your life.

By simply following some of the above tips and by eliminating the source that triggers eczema you can treat eczema naturally and organically via Ayurveda.

Why should you treat eczema using natural and organic products?

Eczema is a skin disease that affects millions of people around the world. This disease causes skin irritation, redness, inflammation and itchiness.

These symptoms appear because of lack or deficiency of nutrients on your body, mainly **Vitamin E** and **Aloe Vera**.

These 2 nutrients are vital for the skin self-defense system. <u>They are the fuel source of the skin self-defense system</u>. Without them the skin self-defense system cannot perform its tasks.

<u>This is the real reason why creams and lotions work well to give instant relief from eczema; they are artificially enhanced with these 2 nutrients.</u>

So my question to you is this, **<u>why would you take these 2 nutrients artificially</u>**?

You can always receive these 2 nutrients naturally! Most vegetables and fruits are organically rich with these 2 nutrients.

Another advantage of eating healthy food is that they are 100% safe with no side effects! **Unlike creams and lotions.**

<u>This is the reason why natural and organic medicine is getting more and more popular these days.</u>

And I really recommend trying natural treatment before going to the ordinary clinical medicine.

Do not get me wrong, clinical medicine works very well! But it is not the safest option in the long run because they are made from chemicals and these <u>chemicals in the long run causes numerous side effects.</u>

Unlike clinical medicine, <u>organic products have no side effects at all because they are made from fruits and vegetables.</u>

And fruits and vegetables are considered healthy food because they are **naturally** enhanced with vital nutrients, vitamins and minerals.

Benefits of Organic Treatments for Eczema

A lot of people are switching from medical medicine to organic medicine and this made me write this article, I will show you the benefits of organic treatment.

Do not get me wrong! I have nothing against medical medicine whatsoever! Medical treatment is very effective; it is based on years and years of studies and experiences. However medical science is very expensive and fairly unsafe, meaning it does cause side effects.

This is what made people in switching from medical treatment into organic treatment. You see organic medicine is composed from natural and organic materials, such as fruits and vegetables. Due to this nature of treatment ingredients, organic medicine does **not cause any sort of side effects!**

What organic treatment tells is that: fruits and vegetables contain high level of vital nutrients for human body. Which is true, fruits and veggies are proven to contain high level of vitamins and minerals.

If you compare **medical medicine over organic medicine**, you will figure it out that they are not that different. In the sense that: what medical medicine does is that it provides those vital nutrients that I just mentioned earlier in a form of creams, lotions or pills. Here these nutrients are artificially made via chemicals and these harsh chemicals **cause side effects**!

Organic treatment on the other hand extract those same vital nutrients but via a more natural way, buy consuming fruits and vegetables and therefore organic medicine does not cause any sort of side effects!

Does organic treatment really work?

Of course it does! Organic medicine is a very ancient medicine, long ago ancient people used plants, flowers, fruits and vegetables to treat and cure several types of disease. Over time these ancient treatments got lost and now people are re-finding these old and ancient organic cures.

And I truly believe that organic medicine is the best medicine for all sorts of human body problems, including eczema. Organic treatment is the safest and most effective way to treat and cure eczema.

Go ahead! Give organic medicine a go and I guarantee you that you will not regret! Stop spending hundreds of dollars in expensive harsh chemicals that cause side effects, stop risking and start living the healthier way! Go organic and be happy!

Total natural way to treat and cure Eczema without risking any sort of side effects!

Eczema disease can strike to anyone at any time! From children, teenagers and adults no one can escape to this awful disease.

How can I get infected with Eczema?

There are numerous ways to get infected with Eczema, if someone of your family had been diagnosed with this disease that chances are that you will also inherit it as well.

However this is not the only way to get infected with Eczema. Allergies such as dust, detergents, fragrances and cloths can easily trigger Eczema.

You see detergents and fragrances contain harsh chemicals that can react very badly especially on people who have sensitive skin. Twenty percent of Eczema patients suffer from this. Therefore if you have sensitive skin then avoids using these sorts of products.

Clothes can also trigger Eczema; this may sound a bit odd. Let me explain, clothes such as wool can also react badly on people who have delicate skin; you see wool is very rough material. And this can easily strike Eczema. So if you are allergic to wool, then I suggest wearing cotton clothes, you see cotton is a very soft, smooth and itchy free material. Studies show that cotton molecules upon direct contact with an Eczema skin provide an instantaneous relief from itchiness and irritation.

The majority of people diagnosed with Eczema suffer from the lack of skin nutrients; this unbalance causes Eczema, which is inevitable.

I have Eczema how do I treat it?

There are loads of creams and lotions out there, and they work great! However not only they are extremely expensive but they also cause numerous side effects. Therefore I believe they are not the ideal solution to fight Eczema.

So what is the best way to treat Eczema?

Remember when I said that the majority of people diagnosed with Eczema suffer from the lack of skin nutrients. Well to prove that I was not lying... I will reveal the secret of creams and lotions.

These medical prescriptions (creams, lotions and pills) are made from artificial chemicals, well everybody knows that! But that sort of chemical are there, do you know?

I will tell you! Eczema creams and lotions contain artificially enhanced skin nutrients, mainly Vitamin E and Aloe Vera.

By applying these creams and lotions to our skin, we are injecting these key nutrients to our skin. However these nutrients are made from harsh chemicals that will definably cause side effects!

So ask yourself! Should I inject artificial nutrients to my skin? Or should I get these key nutrients organically!

How do I get these key nutrients organically?

By eating fruits and vegetables that are naturally rich in these 2 key nutrients, Vitamin E and Aloe Vera!

A total natural and organic way to treat and cure Eczema without risking any sort of side effects!

Treat Eczema Using Household Products, Instead of Medicine

Eczema is a skin disease that affects millions around the world. It is estimated that 1 out of 17 suffers from eczema. And these numbers are rising, which is pretty scary.

But fortunately there is cure for eczema, and I am not talking about pills, lotions or crèmes! I am talking about household products that can treat and cure eczema.

Curing eczema with household products, is it possible?

Yes! It is possible and many people use it with positive results. I will share in this article some of the ways you can treat eczema using this method.

But why should I use household products to cure eczema?

This is a valid question! And the answer is very simple. You see household products that I am talking about are all organic material, meaning they are made from natural products that you consume daily. And because of that it does not have any side effects, unlike medicine.

As you know medicines are made from chemicals and these chemicals cause numerous side effects on the long run. But with organic products this issue is virtually eliminated.

What medicine does is to provoke your body to stimulate chemical reactions that is required to fight any disease.

So how can I treat eczema using organic or household products?

You can treat eczema using household products to stimulate chemical reactions that was motioned earlier, without using medicine but naturally!

You see one of the main causes of eczema is dry skin, and dry skin happens once your body stops producing vitamin E and Aloe Vera.

So instead of consuming these tablets, why don't you consume fruits and vegetables that are rich in these 2 nutrients?

Below is a small list of fruits and vegetables that are rich in vitamin E and Aloe Vera:

· Blackberries
· Avocado
· Plums
· Almonds
· Hazel nuts
· Peanuts
· Broccoli
· Leeks

This is a more healthy and natural approach to cure eczema.

Kill the root source of your Eczema and be Eczema free forever!

I had Eczema and I know how awful and annoying it is, luckily I was able to defeat Eczema and I will teach you exactly how I accomplished this. In this article I will show you the most powerful way to treat and cure eczema, and I am not talking about creams, lotions or pills!

Eczema is a skin disorder that causes severe dryness, itchiness, irritation, inflammation and redness. It is not just a rash, but a severe skin disease that drives you nuts! This skin disorder causes extreme itchiness and irritation; it makes you scratch and scratch all day! I remember how I used to suffer from this awful skin condition. Sometimes I used to scratch so hard that I used to start bleeding, and even so the itchy feeling didn't died away... that is how awful and uncomfortable this disease is.

Like other Eczema patients I tried numerous creams and lotions, I even tried some very expensive ones that cost me over hundred and twenty dollars each! They provided me temporarily relief from these annoying symptoms. However how good these creams and lotions were they never cured my Eczema, meaning the Eczema never stop coming back!

After years of suffering I finally found a cure that kills the source of Eczema, and once the source is killed Eczema is gone forever! And this is what I am going to share with you guys!

So are you ready? The ultimate solution that I found is not creams or lotions, but far more natural and organic. It is called organic treatments for Eczema.

This treatment is based on a combination of pure natural and organic products, such as fruits, vegetables, plants and flowers. Some people even called this homemade medicine for Eczema.

How can fruits, vegetables, plans or even flowers can cure my Eczema?

Fruits, veggies, plans and flowers contain vital nutrients required for a healthy looking skin. You see when the human body suffers from the deficiency of these vital nutrients it reacts, and the result of this reaction is Eczema.

No matter how much you will spend on expensive creams and lotions you will never get cured from Eczema, unless you re-establish the nutrients deficiency of your body and skin. Once the skin fulfils the necessary requirements you will be Eczema free forever!

Eczema - How to Cure the Symptoms Fast

Eczema is an inflammatory and chronic skin disorder. Due to loss of moisturizer the skin becomes dry, red or pink in color, patches occur with scaly skin, blisters bump up filled with pus in acute cases. The skin becomes available for the bacteria and viruses to get penetration without any protection.

Following are some natural methods to cure the symptoms fast based on diet:

The acute Eczema can be cured with cold wet fomentation and cold compress. It should be wrapped with some thick and soft cloth. The cloth to be wrapped must be wet with cold water which is 55-60 degree Fahrenheit. It should be changes after every 15 to 30minutes. It is a temporary relief method.

The best way is to cleanse the body and the blood stream completely. The best thing is to drink orange juice and water regularly in high dozes for about 5-10 days as per the severity of the problem. It is better to say to fast on juice and water.

After the juice fast eat lots of fruits, steamed veggies, raw veggies and salt free food items along with chapattis and whole meal bread. Carrots and musk melon are the best. Instead of ghee make use of coconut oil.

Eat loads of sprouts along with yeast, honey and vegetable oils. Try to add the juice fast after a month or two.

It is recommended to avoid high flavored food items, alcoholic beverages, coffee and tea. Also prevent the use of tinned food, denatured cereals like pearled barley, polished rice, white flour products, and sugar. Eat only wholesome and pure foods.

Other methods to cure the symptoms fast:

- The person affected with eczema should get fresh air as much as possible.
- Coconut oil to be applied on to the affected areas of the skin.
- Jogging and walking should be recurred to activate the bowels.
- Have sun bath to destroy the bacteria.

Skin dryness? Moisturize your skin without creams and lotions

Eczema is a skin disorder that causes numerous symptoms such as itchiness, dryness, irritation, inflammation and sometimes bleeding. This skin disease is more common on young children however recent studies suggest that adults are also very vulnerable.

Why do you need to moisturize your skin?

As mentioned earlier eczema causes dryness therefore moisturizing your skin is always a good idea. Creams and lotions do work, but most of them cause numerous side effects! Therefore they are not the best solution for skin dryness.

Is there a better way to moisturize your skin? With zero risk of side effects?

The answer is YES! There is a better way, a more natural way moisturize your skin and it guarantees zero side effects! So what is it? **Water!** Yes you have heard right, water is a natural moisturizer and by drinking 2 to 3 liters of water a day and taking daily showers your will not only moisturize your body and skin but you will also prevent dehydration.

And what is great about this is that there are no side effects! And water is much cheaper than buying expensive moisturizing product such as creams and lotions. So ask yourselves, why spend hundreds of dollars in these expensive products and risk side effects? Why not do it the natural way!

Beat your itching problem for ever: common causes of itching

Itching can be induced by a number of conditions, but the most common is **Eczema**. There are a numerous creams, lotions and medications to get temporarily relief from the itchiness of Eczema. But these medications are very expensive, and they have numerous side effects and if that wasn't enough, some do not even work! This leaves those suffering from severe itching wondering what really does?!

What is the cause of Eczema?
The first step towards treating eczema (itchiness) is to learn more about what causes the itch, it can be allergy related eczema, such as diet, detergent or any other medical condition.

Trying a new shampoo or soap can lead to eczema as they are made from harsh chemicals that can react badly to an allergic skin. Not only that your diet can also induce Eczema. Nut allergy is a very common disease that triggers eczema.

Some of the most common factors that cause eczema are fabric softeners, fatty foods, caffeine, and certain types of materials. It is a good idea to take these into consideration as well as laundry detergent and other cleansing products.

Hydrate your skin to cure Eczema
Water will flush out all the toxins that build up in the bloodstream of your body. These toxins often lead to conditions that cause symptoms such as itching. Water hydrates the skin, allowing the body to naturally moisturize therefore reducing itching, dryness and even cracking that are associated with the itching.

So there you go, some of the most common causes that triggers itching and how to beat it naturally!

What Makes Eczema Spread Fast?

Eczema as most of you know is a skin disorder that causes numerous symptoms but the most common are: skin rash, reddish pigments on the surface of the skin, itchiness, inflammation and sometimes bleeding.

This disease is common on young children, but recent studies shows that adults are also being diagnosed with eczema.

What makes this disease stand out from the others skin disorders is that it can spread very fast throughout your body in a matter of days.

But what causes this spreading? And more importantly how to stop?!

A lot of people ask me these 2 questions very frequently and I can understand why, eczema is very annoying feeling and does cause discomfort, especially when you are in public. The itchy feeling is so intense that leaves you no choice but to scratch, scratch and scratch!

Sometimes is scratching act goes far as bleeding, and even so it does not satisfy your feeling of scratching. This is what eczema is, a very annoying itchy disease.

Now let's get back to the original question, what causes the quick spreading of the disease?

The answer is, scratching! Yes, I know what you are thinking, if that is the reason then there is no solution, because the itchy felling is so intuitive and leaves you no choice but to scratch, right?

Wrong! No matter what the disease makes you do, avoid scratching, this act will multiply the disease faster and it will spread throughout your body before you know it!

So what is the solution?

The solution is to apply Natralia Eczema & Psoriasis Cream, this cream will kill the eczema bacteria's and prevent them to never come back, giving you an itchy free life forever!

I had eczema for years and usual medications didn't help. Until I found Natralia Eczema & Psoriasis Cream, after applying this cream the disease disappeared in a few days! My skin has been healthy ever since.

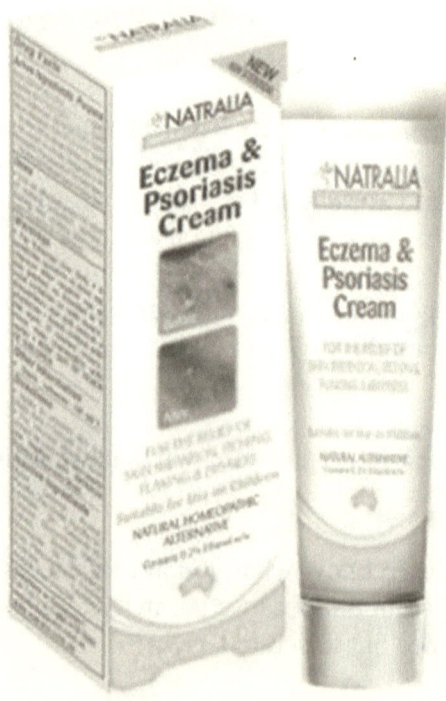

Natralia Eczema and Psoriasis Cream (2oz)

Natralia Eczema and Psoriasis Cream (2oz) - The Best Cream over the Counter - Here is a Review

There are hundreds of Eczema creams and lotions over the counter, but Natralia Eczema and Psoriasis Cream is without a doubt the best of them all! This product is made from pure organic materials such as: herbs and essential oils that provides a soothing relief from rash symptoms.

Unlike other lotions out there Natralia is proved to have virtually no side effects. Natural and organic ingredients mentioned earlier are the key for this. This is one of many reasons why Natralia is so popular!

Natralia works as a moisturizer that provides instantaneous relief from skin rash; its secret formula not only eases the Eczema symptoms but gradually kills it, upon regular use.

This product really works tacking every single skin conditions; this is the reason why skin specialist recommends Natralia Eczema and Psoriasis Cream.

This cream is also suitable for young children.

Unlike other creams and lotions, Natralia can be applied on the face and thought the body. So you do not require to buy any another Eczema facial lotion, Natralia does it all!

As you know Eczema generally spreads fast when it comes to direct contact with soaps and detergents. Due its harsh chemicals that irritate skin disorder, luckily there is Natralia Eczema and Psoriasis Wash. This works just like regular soap, but with without harsh chemicals, instead it has an added mild Natralia secret formula that reduces rash symptoms while you wash your skin.

Natralia is without a doubt the best formula to treat every single Eczema symptoms.

PIH, UV Rays and Eczema

When you've eczema, post inflammatory hyper pigmentation draws some areas of your skin appear darker than other areas do. The dimmed areas likewise tend to suffer pigments that can make the skin appear like a type of fungus is developing on it. Whenever you discover yourself distressed with PIH, recognize that it's a long procedure, but it's likely that the events of PIH can be revoked. Here are 2 simple steps that you are able to use to shrink your chances of being bothered with PIH.

PIH reproduce once the melanin cells in the skin get mutilated as an act of inflammation. It was likely that the inflammation was alleged to go to the position of a problem, repair the problem and then leave. Occasionally it doesn't behave that way. Some of the times the inflammation attends the site of an insult, and adjusts the problem but then carries on to process in the area even though there's no problem to solve. Once this happens, organs (in our example the skin,) can get mutilated.

To forbid this from occurring you are able to reduce your factors of inflammation. PIH is mainly an inflammation based problem. Once you cut down inflammation, it's plausible that PIH won't run out of control and induce these types of problems.

You'll likewise want to keep out of the sun. Direct exposure to sunlight is believably the most cogent promoter of inflammation out of all. UV rays have the power to rapidly expand inflammation, making PIH more approachable as a side effect of oxidization and inflammation burning.

This is way Sun creams is vital to use when you go to the beach, these types of creams create a thin barrier to protect your skin and prevent skin burns. These types of creams can also be beneficial for eczema sufferers because eczema has been proven to inflame when the diseased skin is in direct contact with the Sun as mentioned earlier in this article.

Find Why Acidity Can Cause Eczema - How to Cure Acidy Eczema Symptoms

Eczema and acidity, this may sound new to you, but the fact is that 20% of eczema suffers are caused by acidity. The reason is simple, high level acidity causes changes on your body and eczema occurs as a symptom.

Let me in detail what really happens and what strikes eczema.

You see on our daily lifestyle we consume lots of products that are acid rich, such as sugars, carbohydrates, excess fats and uric acid (all very common in our modern diets) keep flowing through our bloodstream. All these excess acids reacts with the body balance, what it means is that body is trying to neutralize the acids, but because the acids are overflowed, your skin gets the glumes of body reaction and hence eczema strikes.

So here comes the exciting part, the cure. To be able to deal with these excess acids on your body you need to cleanse it. Cleansing your body will remove the excess acids and you will see your eczema healing naturally.

So, if you have eczema but you also have acidity, then you should start working on getting relief from acidity first, because this is the root of your eczema. Once the root is killed eczema will die as well.

Although, cleansing your body is a must, but another way to get relief from acidity and eczema is to drink lots of water, because water will dilute the acids and this will help the body to observe the excess acids.

Water and Eczema - Couple of Ways to Treat and Avoid Eczema Quick Spread!

Eczema is a skin disease that causes itchiness, dryness, irritation and inflammation. This skin condition is very common among young teenagers however recent studies show that adults are also very vulnerable.

In this article I will share 2 effective ways to avoid and treat eczema without any sort of medications. The tips shared in this article are totally safe to use and very effective in getting rid of eczema problems.

I used to have eczema and I know how irritating it can be this is why I am writing this article, from my experience I found 2 very effective ways to get priceless relief from its annoying symptoms and they are:

#1 water: water is a natural body moisturizer, believe it or not but by drinking 2/3 liters of water a day you will notice a great relief from itchiness and redness of eczema. I also recommend taking daily showers in order to maintain your body moist and dry free. This will also prevent dehydration.

#2 avoid fragrances: perfumes and aftershaves contain harsh chemicals that reacts very badly with eczema. Believe it or not but fragrances are the main cooperatives for a quick spread of the disease, therefore if you do not want your eczema to spread all over your body then I highly recommend to stop applying perfumes and aftershaves to your skin immediately!

There you go couple of ways to avoid eczema; as you see you do not require any sort of creams, lotions or pills to cure your eczema problems. You can treat it organically by simply drinking 2/3 liters of water a day and of course by avoiding fragrances.

7 Things to Avoid While Suffering From Eczema

In this article I will show you 7 things to avoid while suffering from severe eczema. By simply avoiding these 7 things that I will reveal in this article you will be able to prevent your eczema or even give a full stop for its quick spreading.

Eczema as you know is a very annoying and uncomfortable skin disease; it causes severe itchiness, dryness, irritation, inflammation, redness and sometimes bleeding. This awful disease affects millions around the globe; recent studies suggest that there are 34 million dermatitis patients around the world. And these numbers are rising every year.

There are hundreds of creams, lotions and pills to reduce eczema; along with hundreds of natural and organic cures however these cures will be ineffective or should I say they will provide minimum results unless you avoid certain things that make eczema to multiply and spread quickly. And this is what I am going to reveal in this article, 7 things to avoid the quick spread of eczema.

#1 avoid detergents: detergents are made from harsh chemicals, studies show that direct contact from these harsh chemicals strives eczema to multiply and to spread quickly throughout the body.

#2 avoid fragrances: perfumes, aftershaves, colognes, etc. Also contains harsh chemicals therefore avoid them while you are suffering from eczema.

#3 avoid dairy products: studies suggest that consumption of dairy products such as milk, yogurt somehow irritates damaged skin cells (eczema). Therefore I suggest instead of consuming dairy milk try soya milk for a change.

#4 avoid tanning: tanning you skin while suffering from eczema is not a good idea.

#5 avoid wool cloths: wool clothes are very itchy materials especially when you are suffering from eczema, studies show that wool will cause you 3 times more skin irritation and itchiness, therefore I suggest wearing cotton clothes. Cotton unlike wool will ease these symptoms.

#6 avoid allergic foods/products: this seems obvious you should always avoid things that are allergic to you, however sometimes certain foods or products gets really tempting, but however tempting they can be simply avoid them, it is not a good idea. Once you are eczema free fell free to enjoy them cautiously!

#7 avoid scratching: this is the hardest thing to avoid, I know itchy eczema can be and I know how hard it is to not to scratch but please **do not scratch!** Scratching may give you temporarily relief from it, however by simply scratching you will multiply your eczema in an instant and sometimes scratching can lead in to bleeding. This is the source of the quick spread of eczema, so please no matter how itchy you will **do not scratch!**

Fruits and Vegetables That Heal Eczema - Eczema Organic - Natural Treatment

Did you know that one third of eczema suffers are cause by nutrient deficiencies? Lack nutrients can strike skin eczema. The reason is simple; our skin needs nutrients, so it can remain smooth and healthy.

When the skin finds hard to receive vital nutrients, the skin self-defense system cannot perform their task and as a result, eczema starts.

You see our skin self-defense system, need some kind of energy to work, just like cars needs petrol to run. And how do we get those nutrients? By eating of course!

So you see our skin requires nutrients, but only 2 are vital for our skin defense systems and they are:

- Vitamin E
- Aloe Vera

If you have eczema them you are probably using creams to relief from itching, but did you ever wondered why creams works so well? Let me tell you why! The reason is that these creams are enforced with these 2 vital nutrients artificially!

So why expending hundreds on artificial products to cure eczema if you can cure it naturally by consuming natural and organic products such as fruits and vegetables! And fruits and vegetables as you know are very healthy products. Many people tried this healthy approach and they successfully got relief from eczema forever! This approach is getting more and more popular and day by day people are filling more healthy and itchy free.

Below are some of the fruits and vegetables example that you should eat to get relief from eczema, as they are rich in vitamin E and Aloe Vera, they are:

- Blackberries
- Avocado
- Plums
- Almonds
- Hazel nuts
- Peanuts
- Broccoli
- Leeks
- Spinach
- Potato

Why Does Epsom Salt Bath Treatment Works to Reduce Eczema?

An Epsom salt bath is rich in magnesium which is essential for your body, as this helps to eliminate all the harmful acids on your skin. Also by taking this bath and soaking yourself will reduce your muscular pain and alleviate your body stress, making it something like a spa bath.

There are a lot of bathing recipes online that makes use of Epsom salts. Some of these recipes even include essential oils for added aromatherapy. You must always remember that eczema is often attributed to skin dryness, and that's what you have to avoid. Also note, do not use any kind of soap when taking an Epsom salt bath or else it would obstruct the healing action of the salts. You can soak in for about 15 minutes and gently give your skin a good gentle rub.

Although this bath is very helpful to moisture your skin and eliminate all the unwanted skin enzymes, this alone is not enough to cure eczema. Along with this Epsom salty bath treatment you must also follow a good diet of fruits and vegetables that are rich in Vitamin E and Aloe Vera. These 2 ingredients are essential for a healthy looking skin, as they are responsible for the skin defense system. Without them we cannot win the battle against Eczema.

Alcohol and Eczema

Eczema is a skin disease that causes dry skin which often results in an itchy and irritating skin. And one of the reasons for this disease to strike is dehydration. So if you drink lots of alcoholic drinks and you have eczema, this can be one of the many causes why you suffer from this skin disease. You see, alcohol is proven to dehydrate your body which also includes human skin. Not only that but it is also known that massive consumption of alcohol can lead to more severe and lethal diseases such as cancer.

The best alternative is to drink water, about 2/3 litters a day, this will ensure that your body is hydrated and your skin will fill more moisturize, because water is flowing in your body. And water is also low in calories, and can easily fill up your stomach and help you to lose weight if you drink it in a proper time and in a proper way (just before taking a meal).

Also to be noted, not to drink high amount of caffeine, if you are infected with eczema. Caffeine is also proven to react very badly with the disease, this can cause a rapid spread of eczema, so reduce the amount to caffeine a day. I suggest no to drink more then 2 cups of coffee a day if you want to reduce eczema more quickly.

Also I suggest eating lots of fruits and vegetables, because they are naturally rich in water as well as in vitamins and minerals. Vitamin E and Aloe Vera are 2 vital nutrients for your skin self defence system, so eat as many fruits and vegetables as you can, this is ensure that your skin receives the right amount of key nutrients and your skin will be healthy in no time.

Eczema Alternatives Treatment - How to Use Grape Seed Oil to Cure and Relief from Eczema

Eczema as you know is a skin disease that causes itchiness, irritating and sometimes bleeding. All this symptoms often leaves scars, red spots and harsh surface.

Luckily there are many natural cures that beliefs the pain on eczema. One of which is the use of **grape seed oil**.

Why Grape Seed Oil?
Because of its properties, it had abilities to recreate cells that were attacked from eczema disease. Not only that but also grape seed oil a natural skin moisturizer.

Grape seed oil cleanses the body from harmful radicals and it also increases blood circulation. That is why this oil is well known as an antidote to reduce inflammation and irritation of skin related diseases.

So you see grape seed oil can relief you from eczema symptoms. It will ease the pain and relief from irritating and inflammation of the diseased skin.

So if you want an alternative treatment for curing and relieving from eczema, grape seed oil is certainly one of the ways to do it.

Let me also give you some more tips and advice to that will prevent eczema to strike again.

First of all if you used to wear wool cloths, stop immediately! Wool is an excellent conductor that reacts with eczema skin. Wool creates a passage way to the eczema to multiply, this will make your skin radish and irritated. Instead wear cotton wear, cotton is a soft cloth and warm as well. Cotton doesn't react at all with eczema.

Also if you suffer from eczema try to moisturize your skin as often possible. Moisturizing is very important during eczema, because it cleans the skin and eliminates all the bad bacteria and allows an easy passage way to the self-defense system to work properly.

Oatmeal to Cure Your Eczema - The Secret Recipe Finally Revealed!

In this article I will share the magic properties of oatmeal that will cure your Eczema problems without any sort of prescriptions! A totally natural and organic way to treat Eczema without risking side effects!

Eczema as you know is a skin disease that causes itchiness, redness, irritation, inflammation and dryness. This skin condition is very common among young children although recent studies suggest that adults are also vulnerable.

In this article I will share a natural ingredient that will change your life! No more itching, swelling and defiantly no more embarrassment.

Forget creams, lotions and pills. You do not require prescription drugs to treat your Eczema. Not only they are expensive but they also cause side effects! What you need is a solution that will cause zero side effects and it is made from natural ingredients.

And below is your answer!

Oatmeal Paste

Mix oatmeal with water and create a paste and apply it over your Eczema skin. And leave it for about 20 minutes or so afterwards you may wash it with water. This paste will act as your pharmaceutical cream and will provide priceless relief from the most annoying Eczema symptoms!

This really works! And it is made from a natural ingredient, a totally natural and organic way to treat Eczema! And by being organic is causes zero side effects! Give it a go today, do it for at least a week and you will notice amazing results! Oatmeal Past the best homemade remedy for Eczema skin.

Raw Honey to Treat Eczema

Raw Honey that can heal your Eczema with zero pain. This is an ancient Eczema recipe that was kept hidden for centuries and finally it's getting revealed!

Eczema as you know is a skin disorder that causes itchiness, redness, irritation, inflammation and dryness. This skin condition has been around for centuries and ancients found a great homemade solution for this awful skin disease.

In this article I will reveal the magic ingredient that will heal your Eczema without any sort of prescriptions, a totally natural and organic treatment for Eczema.

Raw Honey

Yes you have heard right! This ancient ingredient contains magical properties that can heal Eczema. This is what ancients used to do, they used to apply Raw Honey over their diseased skin and leave it from about 20 minutes or so. After that they washed with water.

Recent studies reveal that Raw Honey upon direct contact with Eczema provides a soothing feeling that gives you priceless relief from Eczema symptoms. It works just like your chemist creams, were the actual cream is Honey!

What is great about this ancient homemade therapy is that it does not cause any sort of side effects, unlike prescription drugs and it is a lot cheaper than buying those expensive Eczema creams and lotions.

Keep Eczema Skin Moisturized Without Prescription

There are plenty of ways to moisturize your skin; you do not require creams or lotions. Or any other prescription drugs, in this article I will show you 2 effective ways to moisturize your skin without prescription drugs.

Eczema is a skin disease that causes dryness, itchiness and irritation and therefore moisturizing is a must. There are loads of moisturizing creams out there however not only they are expensive but they also cause side effects.

In this article I will show you couple of ways to moisturize you're without drugs. Below are 2 effective ways to moisturize your skin:

#1 water: water is a natural body moisturizer therefore drinking 2 to 3 litres of water a day and by taking daily showers you will not only moisturize your body and skin but also prevent dehydration. This is a natural and organic way to moisturize your skin and treat Eczema.

#2 Coconut: many people do not know but coconut contain magical moisturizing properties, therefore applying coconut to your skin not only provides a soothing cool feeling but also keeps your skin moist.

Eczema Milk Treatment Recipe

Is your skin fill itchy and irritating?

If the answer of the above questions is Yes! Then you probably have Eczema! And if that is the case then you probably are using creams to moisturize your skin. As these creams are rich in vitamin E and Aloe Vera, which makes you relief from itching.

Although there is nothing wrong on with that treatment, it is proven to work to many people. Vitamin E and Aloe Vera are essential for a healthy skin. And I highly recommend using it!

But as you know these creams can get expensive, and that's why I am writing this article. You see you can create a similar effect to get relief from eczema, using homemade products such as Milk.

Yes Milk. You probably thinking that it is impossible, even doctors suggest avoiding milk so how can milk cure eczema? Well you're right; if you suffer from eczema you should avoid consumption of milk. But what I am going to tell you is something different. You are not going to consume milk orally, but instead using it in a different way.

So are you ready?

To use this treatment you should pour a gallon of whole milk into a tub of lukewarm water and then soak in it. Be careful on this, the water must not to be very hot, because very hot water can activate histamines activity within your skin cells and cause you to itch. So it must be warm water but not hot water.

Now when you are soaking the milk, your skin will absorb the fats that are contained in the milk. These facts are used as moisturizers, just like moisturizers on the creams, and they will strengthen your skin, moistening it and making it more durable and flexible!

Now you must wonder why will these happen, right? Well let me tell you why.

You see Milk contains high amounts of lactic acid and this acid penetrates your skin and that penetration makes you loose and removes dead skin cells that are on the surface of your skin. And when these dead cells are removed, the skin becomes bacterial free and allowing the under skin up and making the skin stronger and younger and better able to protect the body and do the work that skin is supposed to do.

Flax Seeds - Natural Way to Cure Eczema

Eczema can persist, especially if a person is exposed to chemicals which can cause irritation or allergy in a human body. It occurs less often in infants but it is common in adults. The symptoms may be seen in inner elbow and behind the knees.

In Modern world many medicines came into existence for the treatment of eczema. Those medicines are capable to eradicate the eczema completely. But the problem is that they can cause some new disorders in human body. Few researchers found that Flax seeds can be used for the treatment of Eczema. It can be found in any whole seed market or in herbal medicine store.

The main substance that helps to cure eczema is omega 6 and omega 3 fatty acids. Fortunately these fatty acids are found enormously in flax seeds. One great advantage in using this seeds for the treatment of eczema is that it can cure the disorder without any side effects. Also the seeds can be very useful in treating other skin disorder like psoriasis. This is because of the anti-inflammatory property that the flax seed holds.

Treating eczema with flax seeds is very easy, an infected person can take these flax seeds along with meals or cereals in every morning. These people can also take these seeds with water or juice. Also gel made from these seeds can be applied on the surface of the infected region. One can take these seeds for treatment of eczema as pills which are readily available in the health stores.

Herbal extracts from the chamomile, licorice and witch hazel can also be used for the treatment of eczema.

How to Cure Baby Eczema

It is very difficult for parents to realize that their baby is suffering from Baby Eczema! Baby eczema can occur in every part of their body such as flare-up on the forehead, scalp, and chest and nearby area of the joints. And if left untreated, it can turn out to be extremely itchy and inflamed and the babies may experience long sleepless nights.

Causes There are many causes to Baby Eczema but the most common one is the hereditary cause. Parents or a relative who had or currently have eczema then it is likely that their baby will get it as well. Other cause can be from an allergic reaction such as carpet or any other allergic reaction.

Treatment Baby eczema treatment plan involves a wide array of remedies that can effectively improve the skin condition of the baby and help in alleviating irritation to some extent. Moisturizing is absolutely essential to avoid itching sensation and to get rid of all discomforts related to the drying skin condition. Bathing baby in lukewarm water can help baby's skin to retain moisturizer. You must not rub the skin of your baby, but pat it to dry.

Doctors suggest mothers to put cotton clothes on their babies. It is highly discouraged to use woolen or synthetic materials, because it worsens the skin condition even more. Keep your child in a dust-free environment. Although pets can be a good playing partner for your kids, but their hair can cause allergies and skin irritation for your child. So keep pets away from your baby, especially if he or she is suffering from baby eczema.

Babies and Eczema - 3 Things to Avoid

Eczema generally triggers upon dry skin but there are other ways to get infected with Eczema, such as: lotions, detergents and diet.

Babies tend to spend a lot of time with their mother, if you are a mother then be careful. Do not use strong fragrances or makeup. These can easily trigger Eczema to your children; these kinds of products contain harsh chemicals that react very badly on young skin. Most parents unaware of this.

Also be very careful in choosing detergents such as soaps. The young one love to take baths, certain types of soap can easily strike Eczema. Make sure that your children skin is not sensitive, most soap will have the chemical components written on the side; make sure that it does not contain harsh chemicals as they will react very badly on young skin.

Babies and children tend to have a great milky diet, believe it or not but dairy products in some rare cases can trigger Eczema, simply because they contain numerous enzymes. In some rare cases those enzymes can cause an allergic reaction which can trigger Eczema.

So there you go 3 things to avoid: fragrances (perfumes and makeup), detergents (soaps) and in daily products (in some rare cases). Avoid these things and reduce the chances of Eczema in your children. Keep your babies safe and healthy.

Avoid Food That Causes Eczema

Eczema is a skin disorder that affects millions of people worldwide every year. It is generally caused by inflammation. Though it is an inherited disease, there are also other factors that cause eczema. The skin becomes very dry producing blisters resulting in itching and burning of the skin. Eczema is commonly seen in hands, arms, wrist, neck, legs and face.

Though there are many potential causes for this skin disease, many people do not realize the fact that eczema is also caused by the food they consume on daily basis. Whenever you are allergic to certain substances you must take care of your diet. This is to prevent the food causing allergies from triggering the development of Eczema. Allergies to smoke, detergents, dust may also cause Eczema but most often it is caused by allergic food substances.

To prevent Eczema caused by allergic food items, you must know them well. So, what are the foods that can cause Eczema?

- Dairy/milk products
- caffeine
- Eggs
- Wheat
- Acidic fruits
- Nuts and red meat
- Sea food
- Chemical food additives like the
    - Tartrazine
    - Sodium Benzoate
    - Sodium glutamate
    - Sodium metabisulphate
- Preservatives

Nutritional deficiencies including deficiency of vitamin B6 also count to the factors causing Eczema It is wise to avoid the above food items in the diet to protect you from Eczema. Drink as much as possible amount of water daily to replace the moisture content of the skin.

Anyone who is affected by Eczema is bound to cut down these food stuffs from the daily diet though they are not allergic to any of these items. To reduce the occurrence of Eczema, it is necessary for an individual to maintain a healthy diet that is balanced and focused on the guidelines put forth by the food pyramid.

Eczema Solution

I Love to speak to you about the eczema solution. There are a lot of people that suffer from this problem. I used to have it for several years before I ever worked out how to resolve the problem. If you are unknown with it, it leaves a dry reddish surface area on your skin. It can be really itchy and occasionally very irritated.

I had it on my cheek right below my eyes and on my brow. It gave this really ugly look to the skin that I did not wish people to see. After years of not acknowledging what to do about it, I discovered a solution that worked great. I am going to share with you the eczema solution.

Among the most common things folks inquire me about my condition is "why do not you just go to a doctor and get it fixed conclusively?" My answer is simply, "I already have". I did go to my doctor and he did analyzed the reddish pique on my face only to conclude that it was not eczema. He told me to get a particular cream and it never worked.

At this point I had to find another way to resolve this problem as the doctor did not know what he was talking about.

The eczema solution is truly simple. Most people think it's a topical solution that requires creams, but it really isn't. You need to get more dietary fat into your diet, essentially the fatty acids (EFA). I started to take some tablespoonful of extra virgin olive oil daily and after about a week my eczema was virtually gone.

Eat the Right Food to Cure Eczema Naturally

Eczema can strikes on babies, children and adults. Recently babies aged little as 2 years were found with severe Eczema.

What strikes Eczema?!

This is the most common and frequent question asked by people. So let me tell you what drives eczema to strike.

There are many reasons, why but the most popular is:

-   Lack of nutrients

Lack of nutrients, this is the most common cause to eczema to strike. And what are the nutrients, you may ask. There are mainly 2 types of nutrients, that your skin self-defense system requires performing their tasked, as these are:

-   Vitamin E
-   Aloe Vera

This to nutrients are vital for the skin defense system, they are the power supply, the fuel or whatever you want to call it. They act like petrol to your car, once the tank is empty your car will stop, just like your skin defense system. If your body skin cannot observe or obtain necessary vitamin E and Aloe Vera, the skin defense will not work. And once the skin defense system is cracked, Eczema can penetrate very easily.

So the solution for this problem is...

Consume lots of food that are rich in vitamin E and Aloe Vera!

Did you why doctors prescribe creams to moisturize your skin when you are suffering from Eczema?

There is because those creams are artificially enhanced with Vitamin E and Aloe Vera! This is why those creams work so well in healing eczema.

So why purchase those expensive creams to treat your eczema, if you can do it naturally, by simple eating food that are naturally rich in Vitamin E and Aloe Vera!

How to Prevent Eczema from Forming

In this article I will reveal how you can prevent eczema from forming! Eczema affects 34 million people around the world and this is why I am writing this informative article. Here I will reveal 5 ways you can prevent and maybe cure your skin dermatitis.

Eczema as you may know is a skin disease that causes severe itchiness, dryness, irritation, inflammation, redness and sometimes bleeding.

There are several ways to get infected by this awful disease; you can get infected via family inheritance (meaning if a direct family member is or was diagnosed with dermatitis you are an ideal candidate to inherit it). You can also catch eczema due to lack of vital nutrients and finally eczema can strike due to dust, pets and other possible allergic reactions.

How do I prevent eczema from forming?

You can prevent or even treat eczema by starting a healthy diet. Eating healthy foods, especially those that are rich in vitamin E and Aloe Vera; since these 2 nutrients are the key for a healthy and smooth human skin. Therefore by having a healthy diet of these nutrients you will prevent or even cure your current eczema.

Wearing cotton clothes is also advisable in order to prevent dermatitis, since cotton is a very smooth, soft and itchy free material. By wearing cotton wear you will reduce skin irritation and therefore prevent eczema.

Drinking 2/3 liters of water a day will prevent dehydration and dry skin. Dryness is one source and symptom of skin dermatitis therefore moisturizing and hydrating your body and skin is always a good idea.

Studies suggest that dairy products conduct eczema, and therefore they to consume minimum amount of these milky products. If you can, switch to soya milk.

Avoid fragrances, perfumes, aftershaves, colognes and any other product that is made from harsh chemicals. These harsh chemicals can react very badly, especially if you have a sensitive skin, and formulate or should I say open the doors for eczema to appear.

How to do if I already have eczema?
If you already got eczema then my advice is try not to scratch yourself! This simple act may give you temporarily relief however what you are actually doing is multiplying eczema and making them to spread quickly over your entire body. So no matter how itchy, irritation or tempting you feel **do not scratch!** If you do you are going 10 steps behind your ultimate goal of curing eczema.

3 best over the counter creams for eczema

Eczema is a skin condition that suffers from itchiness, irritation, inflammation, redness and dryness. There are lots of creams over the counter for this particular skin disorder, but which one is the best? Find out in this article the best performing cream to fight eczema symptoms.

Rash is a very common problem worldwide, it is estimated that there are over 125 million people around the globe with rash and nearly 34 million of them suffers from eczema.

There are literally hundreds of creams and lotions to treat this skin condition, to find which one is the best for you can be tricky. Below are 3 creams that we think are the best creams to fight eczema:

Natralia's Eczema & Psoriasis Cream 2oz

This cream is made from essential oils and natural herbs. This moisturizing cream provides substantial relief from extreme dryness, itchiness and irritation. Unlike other creams this one can be used on the face and all throughout the body. Although there is Natralia Eczema & Psoriasis Wash, soap with mild portion of magical oils that eases eczema symptoms around the face.

Clear Skin-E Eczema Cream

This one is made from pure natural herbs that provide soothing relief from flaky, scaly, itchy, dry and red skin. With a regular use of this cream you will prevent infection, bleeding, cracked skin and also scarring skin. And you eczema scalps will gradually disappear.

Peaceful Mountain's Eczema Rescue Gel 1.0oz

This gel is formulated with herbal oils that provide soothing results. It reduces the rash symptoms and it can also be used for anti-viral/anti-fungal purposes.